This book contains two book manuscripts authored by Sammy Parker:

Book 1: Depression: Naturally Free Yourself of Depression and Heal Anxiety, Panic Attacks, and Stress

Book 2: Charisma: Unshackle your True Charismatic Self and Improve your Social and People Skills. Be a More Confident, Charming, and Charismatic Person

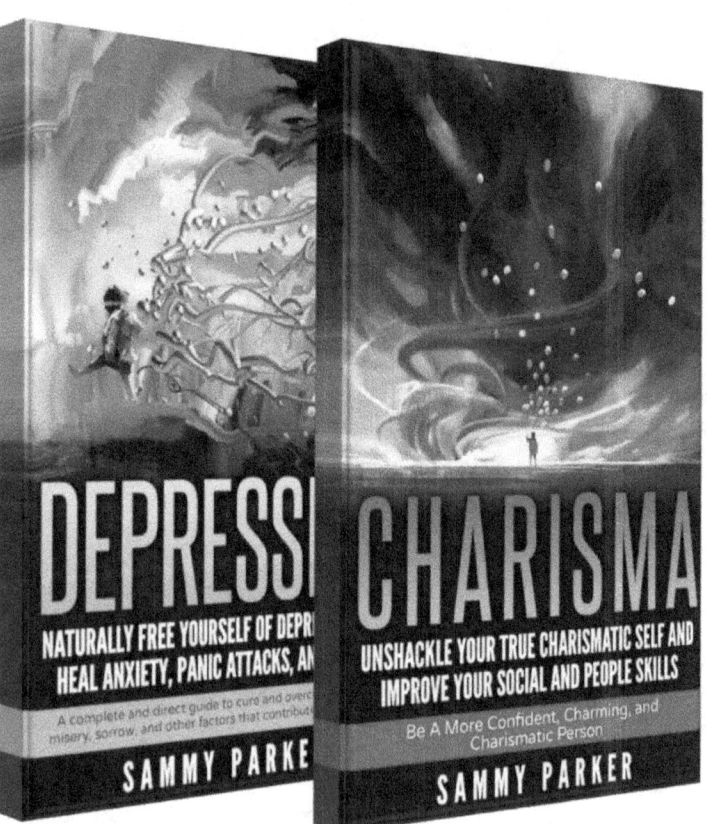

DEPRESSI...

NATURALLY FREE YOURSELF OF DEPR...
HEAL ANXIETY, PANIC ATTACKS, AN...

A complete and direct guide to cure and overc...
misery, sorrow, and other factors that contribute...

SAMMY PARKE...

CHARISMA

UNSHACKLE YOUR TRUE CHARISMATIC SELF AND
IMPROVE YOUR SOCIAL AND PEOPLE SKILLS

Be A More Confident, Charming, and
Charismatic Person

SAMMY PARKER

Depression: Naturally Free Yourself of Depression and Heal Anxiety, Panic Attacks, and Stress

A Complete and Direct Guide to Cure and Overcome Sadness, Misery, Sorrow and Other Factors that Contribute to Depression

BY SAMMY PARKER

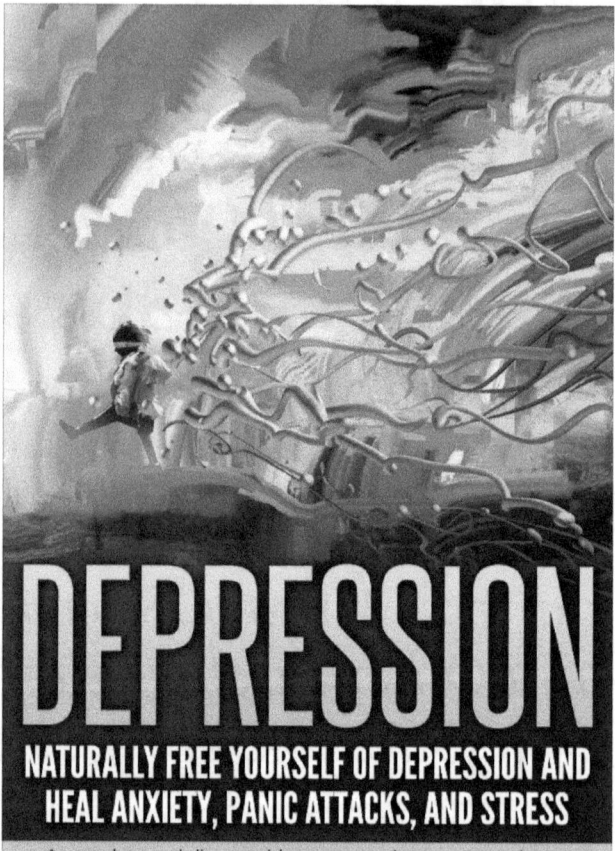

DEPRESSION

NATURALLY FREE YOURSELF OF DEPRESSION AND HEAL ANXIETY, PANIC ATTACKS, AND STRESS

A complete and direct guide to cure and overcome sadness, misery, sorrow, and other factors that contribute to depression

SAMMY PARKER

Preview of this book

Depression can encompass feelings that can include sorrow, misery, sadness, anger, lethargy, and many more. These feelings are related to a disorder, sometimes even a disease or illness within your body.

You are also going to gain insight into the myths of depression. There are common misconceptions that hinder your treatment, as well as do's and don'ts that might be stopping you from gaining proper treatment.

Uncover:

1. How depression affects your life

2. How to boost your self-esteem

3. A care plan to start taking action

4. New discovered, researched, and proven techniques

You are going to discover who the best person to help you will be, so that you can find fulfillment in your life. You might be surprised at who can truly help you the most. Take the journey now. Start your recovery and battle with depression today.

Table of Contents for Depression: Naturally Free Yourself of Depression and Heal Anxiety, Panic Attacks, and Stress

Introduction

Depression affects an estimated 350 people worldwide. People of all ages suffer from depression, including children and retired adults. Depression is also considered the leading cause behind disability on a global scale. Statistics from the World Health Organization show that fewer men suffer depression versus men. Depression can lead to suicide, unless someone seeks the help they need or helps their loved one get the help they need.

Depression is a chronic condition, with long-lasting or severely intense negative emotions. Depression can lead to additional health conditions. It is also a condition that can greatly affect your work, school, and relationships.

More than 800,000 people die each year as a result of suicide, driven by depressive emotions. Suicide due to depression is the second highest cause of death in 15 to 29 year olds, according to the World Health Organization (2016).

If you are one of the 350 million people who suffer from depression, you now know that you are not alone. You have a medical and psychological condition that can be managed with various treatment plans.

You have to be willing to get the help you need or help your loved one see that they can get the treatment they need. There are barriers to proper treatment. It resides in the improper health care system throughout the world, even in developed countries.

A World Health Assembly met in 2013 to focus on the rise of depression among people in the world. This assembly has opened up new pathways for you to gain the treatment and help you need. Many states are now offering free visits to psychologists for low income families. Health insurance has started to add treatment for depression, at least on a minimal basis.

Whether you are a teenager or a senior citizen, you also have tools at your disposal to gain the help you require. This complete and direct guide will help you cure your depression, overcome your anxiety and stress, and get rid of the sadness you feel.

You will be able to have healthy relationships, built on self-confidence, as well as regain your health. Discover what you can do to heal yourself, as well as gain help from others to help you heal. You never know what resources are going to be available to you, until you try.

You are a strong person. You are capable of healing your mind. Take action now and discover how you can eliminate your depression.

I want you to take special attention to chapter 8. This chapter is important because it provides up to date research and techniques that can be used to treat your depression. The main goal of this book is to not only help you understand why you have depression, but also give you a new and holistic views and ideas that are currently present within the past 3 years. I hope this book provides a ton of value to your life and to the lives of others. Thank you!

Chapter 1: Historical View of Depression

Depression is not a new disorder. Historical documents provide us with a pattern of evidence suggesting that depression has always been a health issue for humans. Healers, writers, and philosophers have written about depression, the struggles people have gone through, and ways to treat the illness.

In these historical documents, depression was referred to as melancholia. The first known, written, reference to this disorder was from a 2nd millennium BC Mesopotamian text. During the early centuries, and to a certain degree now, depression and other mental disorders were thought to be demonic possession, thus priests would attend to the "victims" of the disorder.

Physical injuries were handled by physicians, but depression was not considered a physical illness. It was thought of as a spiritual illness. Greek and Roman doctors in later centuries began to think of depression as a biological and psychological disorder. These doctors started prescribing massage, gymnastics, music, special diets, and baths as a cure. They also included a concoction with donkey's milk and poppy extract.

Hippocrates was one of the most famous physicians who attribute depression to personality traits and mental illness as an imbalance of the body fluids. At the time he believed it was an imbalance of black bile, yellow bile, blood, and phlegm. Hippocrates listed mania, phrenitis, and melancholia as mental illnesses. Phrenitis was a brain fever. Hippocrates was the doctor who prescribed bloodletting as a way to treat the imbalance of fluids and to heal depression.

Cicero, a Roman philosopher, had a different opinion. Cicero believed melancholia was due to rage, grief, and fear. His opinion was that depression was not physical, but mental.

More Modern Explanations

In more recent centuries, Robert Burton (1621), wrote the Anatomy of Melancholy. He ascribed depression to psychological and social causes. He felt that fear, poverty, and solitude led to depression. His solution was exercise, diet, travel, distraction, cleansers, herbal remedies, bloodletting, music, and marriage.

The 18th and 19th centuries were a larger change in the thoughts of mental illnesses and depression. The "Age of Enlightenment" listed depression as an unchangeable weakness, one that was inherited, and affected people were shunned. In many cases, they were locked away in institutions and forgotten, (Mental Help, 2007).

Psychology and the understanding of depression have come a long way since the early centuries, even since the early 1900s. Even through the 1950s, mental disorders, including depression were not talked about. If someone suffered from a disorder they were either put in an institution or left at home locked away from visitors.

Psychology started taking a more active, research role, in the 60s and 70s. Aaron Beck developed a new theory about depression in the 60s. He stated depression was caused by negative thinking patterns, where one would think about themselves, their future, and the world.

Other research was working on depression as an endogenous or neurotic reaction. As an endogenous condition, a person would suffer from a biological condition that caused the signs and symptoms of depression. A neurotic or reactive reaction was caused by stressful events.

It was discovered in the 1950s that a chemical imbalance affected the body and brain, leading to depression. Two chemicals in the body caused the imbalance: reserpine and isoniazid. These two chemicals would alter neurotransmitter levels, bringing depressive symptoms to the forefront.

Further work was conducted, where a separation of bipolar disorder and depression were made. In the mid-1970s, a new term was coined—Major Depressive Disorder (Wikipedia, 2016).

Major Depressive Disorder, along with melancholia are listed in the DSM VI versions. Psychology and doctors are still trying to gain a full understanding of depression; however, most understand it is either a chemical imbalance or psychological disorder brought about my fear and anxiety.

Chapter 2: Discover the Cause of Your Depression

Treatment of depression is only possible, when you have an understanding of the cause of your depression. There are main causes of depression that can bring about a temporary condition or one that lasts for one's lifetime. If you are tired of battling your depression, then seek the advice of a physician and psychologist to determine the root cause.

The following are key factors that may lead to depression:

- Abuse

- Medications

- Personal conflicts

- Death or loss

- Genetics

- Major events

- Social isolation

- Illness

- Substance abuse

- Medical disorders

Abuse

Abuse can be sexual, violence, or mental. When inflicted upon a person that person may begin to feel depressed. They start to lose their self-confidence and self-esteem.

Medications

Specific medications prescribed for health issues, such as high blood pressure, can contain beta-blockers. Reserpine can also be included in certain medications.

Both beta-blockers and reserpine can increase the risk of depression in the person taking the medication.

Personal Conflicts

Personal conflicts among friends, family, and co-workers can lead a person to feel depressed, unable to handle the disputes, and unable to face their life.

Death or Loss

The loss of a loved one naturally creates feelings of depression. These feelings can be short lived or may require additional help. It is a mental situation for the person because of their emotions.

Genetics

Studies have found that a family history of depression may link to reserpine and other chemical imbalances, thus a cause can be one's genetic makeup. Depression does not have to link with a genetic disorder for a steady family history of the illness. It can also be linked to the imprinting on the child. A young child may grow up with depression because their main character suffers from it. The exact cause of a family history of depression is still unknown, but there are physical and psychological causes researchers have studied.

Major Events

Major events in your life can be a direct cause of your depression. Marriage, moving, losing a job, getting divorced, losing income, retiring, graduating, obtaining a new job, or suffering from combat can lead to depression.

Social Isolation

Social isolation due to another mental illness, physical illness, or other reason can be a cause of depression. If a person feels like an outcast, there is a potential that the person can feel depressed. Moving away from this isolation or the disparaging remarks can often help a person recover.

Substance Abuse

Substance abuse can be a cause of depression or it can be the result of depression. Approximately 30% of people who suffer from substance abuse issues have also been diagnosed with depression, (Medicine Net, n.d.).

Medical Disorders

Illness, such as cancer, can lead to depression. The reaction to the illness, the feeling that life is over, and the medications required to treat the illness have often been the cause of depression in patients.

The following medical disorders are known to cause depression in patients. These disorders are not as likely to be seen as the cause of depression, and yet for millions of people they can be.

Alzheimer's and Dementia

Patients who are diagnosed with a type of dementia are often suffering from depression. Their confidence begins to dwindle as their memory becomes faulty. They also feel unsettled and worried. Fear and anxiety can lead to depressive symptoms. For some, depression may be the first sign of a brain disorder, such as dementia. Dementia and its various forms, is caused by a shrinking of the brain, which affects mood, memory, and overall cognition.

Thyroid

Thyroid, including Grave's Disease, hyper, and hypo thyroid conditions are an imbalance with a person's hormones. The hormones: TSH, T3, and T4 can become over or under produced. When this occurs, the brain function is affected. There can be short-term memory loss and pseudo-dementia symptoms. When the hormones are corrected, the brain returns to normal function, and depression can be eliminated.

Menopause and PMS

Both are hormonal conditions that have been linked to temporary depression. When the hormone production changes a person can start to feel bad about themselves, feel fatigued, and show other signs of depression. A correction of the hormone production alleviates the troubles.

Chapter 3: Signs and Symptoms

Approximately 10 symptoms are common in people with depression. These common symptoms are not all inclusive. You do not need to have all of them to be considered "clinically" depressed. A diagnosis should be made by a mental health professional or your physician.

Symptoms

- Fatigue

- Concentration difficulty

- Guilt

- Worthless or helpless feelings

- Insomnia, excessive sleeping or early-morning wakefulness

- Restlessness

- Irritability

- Loss of interest

- Appetite changes

- Persistent aches and pains, digestive issues

- Anxiousness, sadness, or an empty feeling

- Thoughts of suicide, or an attempt

These symptoms can occur with physical disorders. For example, a person with a thyroid disorder can feel many of these symptoms, but have a root cause based in a hormonal imbalance. Correcting the hormonal imbalance can adjust a person's way of thoughts and "cure" these depressive symptoms.

Issues can also arise from other mental disorders. Anxiousness, irritability, restlessness, and appetite changes have been caused by social anxiety or other fears.

When the majority of these symptoms are present, then depression is usually the diagnosis, but remember to check for underlying causes.

Warning Signs of Depression

A person who is suddenly very calm or happy after being extremely sad, may have depression.

An individual who always thinks about death or is talking about death may suffer from depression.

With clinical depression, the symptoms become worse, with more trouble sleeping, eating, sadness, or a loss of interest and concentration.

Some people with depression take more risks. These risks are usually based on death, such as driving without headlights, hiking without proper equipment, or being in other situations that could lead to an "accidental" death.

Depression can make you lose interest in relationships and those you truly care about.

You may often be making statements about feeling helpless, hopeless, or worthless. Your self-confidence is at an all-time low. You may feel like people are disrespecting you, treating you incorrectly, or that it is your entire fault because you are worth nothing.

Many people show signs of depression and suicidal thoughts, when they get their life in order. They might change their will or tie up loose ends in preparation of dying.

Talk about dying or killing one's self is not always seen, but in the last days before an attempt is made more of this talk happens. Unscheduled visits or calling people that a person loves can be a sign of suicidal thoughts.

Statements, such as "I want out," or "It is better if I was not here," are usually signs of depression, where the person is getting closer to suicide (Webmd, n.d.).

Hiding Symptoms

Depression takes over slowly. Sometimes a person does not realize they suffer from depression, until their loved one points out the numerous changes in their behavior, relating to the above symptoms.

Other individuals are aware that there are problems, but they ignore the issues or think they can deal with it on their own. This type of person is bound to hide their feelings and symptoms until there is truly no possible way to hide them.

It can be easier if the clinical depression is in a mild form or is a result of a known cause like a recent death in the family. It is also possible that the person has hidden their symptoms for many years due to a high level of self-control, yet they have dangerous thoughts.

Observation is one of the best ways for you to determine if a person around you is hiding their depression symptoms.

If you feel you might have depression, there are things you can do. You can start to track your behavior in a journal. If you already write in a journal, back track and see if you have sudden mood shifts or dark thoughts.

Chapter 4: Depression Misconceptions

Depression like many mental illnesses is seen in the wrong light. These misconceptions can hinder you from getting the help you need. It can also make it difficult for you to understand the disease.

Myths

- **Depression and sadness are the same.** Sadness is a symptom of depression; however, you can be sad without being affected by depression. Sadness can result from a deep, powerful memory. When you think of this memory, you can feel sad, but it is not a constant feeling. Depression is a chronic condition, where sadness is just one of the negative emotions swirling in your brain. The feeling also sucks the life out of you, making daily life arduous.

- **Depression is a sign of mental instability/weakness.** There is a stigma attached to all mental illnesses, including depression. Most people decide to remain quiet about their suffering because of the stigma. The truth is, no one asks to feel depressed, sad, and upset. Depression affects people of all social, psychological, and biological types—not just a specific type of person.

- **It occurs because of a traumatic event**. Yes, there are certain events, which can trigger depression. However, not everyone suffering from depression has gone through a traumatic event. Loving a loved one, being in combat, or going through a divorce can lead to depression. There are feelings of remorse, sadness, emptiness, and loneliness for a period of time. These symptoms may last, without help, for months, even years. Yet, they can also be alleviated within a few weeks.

- **It's all in your mind**. Emotional symptoms do result based on feelings; however, insomnia, fatigue, appetite change, chest pains, and chronic muscle aches can also be an issue. Depression is not just a mental situation, but a physical one, when it goes on long enough.

- **Depression is not a real illness**. Depression is not going to fit one treatment plan, but it does not mean it is not a medical condition that does not require treatment. The Mayo Clinic states that hormone imbalances, the brain, and neurotransmitters that are affected by depression make depression a true illness. It affects a person on various levels.

- **Men don't suffer depression**. The thought that a "real" man will not suffer from depression, is yet another myth. Anyone can be affected by depression. Yes, studies show more women than men suffer from depression, but men still have a higher rate of suicide due to depressive symptoms than women. A middle-aged white male is more at risk for suicide, according to studies. A reason for this myth, is that men tend to have a different way of expressing the problem and thus depression in men is more easily overlooked.

- **All depression is genetic**. Only 10 to 15 percent of people in the world, with a history of family depression will have depression. While it may be hereditary or at least a learned behavior through childhood, it does not mean that if one or both parents are depressive that you will suffer from the same. You do need to be aware and have your levels checked for a chemical imbalance, but this is for peace of mind versus a high risk of developing depression.

- **Medication is the only cure and you need it all your life**. Medication is not the only way to treat your depression. If you do need medication for your depression, you may not need it your entire life. Medication is a short-term requirement. About 40 percent of people with depression use psychotherapy with great results versus medication. Yes, medication can help improve your moods for a time, but your body can also become used to the same medicine, lowering its effects.

- **Discussing your depression makes it worse**. Kids tend to feel this is true, more than adults. Kids feel if they talk about their depression, their feelings will only become worse because those around them will not understand. Adults can also feel this way or feel that talking does not help because they are forced to admit to all the problems they have. In fact, talking about one's feelings is a way to proactively work on positive reinforcement, versus the negative, destructive feelings that rule when you hide your emotions (Hall, 2014).

Knowing these are myths and what the truths are, you can start to focus on your treatment and combat depression in the best possible way for you. There are some Do's and Don'ts that can help you with your depression that also go along with these myths.

Do's

- You do want to recognize that depression can lead to other health issues.

- You want to take steps to minimize other health issues by eating correctly and exercising often.

- It is necessary to develop a way for you to handle stress.

- Get a medical opinion regarding your symptoms and determine if there is an underlying cause of your depression.

- Do understand that medications are only a small help, and there are better treatment options.

Don'ts

- Don't avoid your feelings. Seek treatment.

- Don't settle. You can gain treatment; you don't have to "live" with your moods.

- Don't treat just the depression, look for other causes and determine if there is something else affecting you.

- Don't let inactivity and listlessness win. Make yourself go for a walk.

- Don't neglect the signs you see in yourself. Speak out.

Writing these do's and don'ts is easy. Pushing yourself to follow them and lead a better life is the hard part, but not impossible.

Nothing is impossible, if you try hard enough to face what ails you. Without following through, you could be placing yourself in more danger. Depression can lead to obesity, diabetes, heart attacks, chronic digestive issues, and suicide. Take step after step and work your way to a depression free life. You can do it.

Chapter 5: How Depression Affects Different Aspects of your Life

Depression not only affects you, but it affects various aspects of your life, including the people you love. Discovering how your life is affected by depression can be one more step towards making improvements and pushing you towards the help you need.

Many times we lose sight of those around us, the love we have for them, and how they can help us, when suffering from depression. Reminding yourself that you do have people who care and they are willing to be "bothered" by your troubles will help you in your treatment.

It is true that you will get into a vortex of limited sight when you are in the midst of depression. This cycle of negative thinking can battle between knowing people will help you if you ask, and being unable to ask. Perhaps you have had thoughts that they will not be able to help you or understand. Maybe, you have tried to reach out, but their own lives are busy and you feel like you are just in the way.

There might be times when you've thought, "I'm always the one to get a hold of that person(s), so obviously they do not care about me." Often the other side to the story is that your friends and family do care, but you are right—they are living their life and sometimes that life is just as bad as yours.

Your friends might be battling their own depression. It's even happened to me. I was suffering greatly from depression brought on by the loss of a loved one, although that loved one was not completely gone, his mind was due to dementia. My friend's said they would be there, but never called. It turned out that one of my friends was suffering from post-partum depression and another had been battling depression for 10 years. All three of us didn't tell each other of our struggles and battles with depression, but tried to keep it all inside. Instead of leaning on those that could help and understand, we all chose to keep it to ourselves and try to deal with it in their own way.

The relationships could have been completely and forever fractured. Some relationships were among the friends because of the depression and mistakes made. For example, one friend lost their spouse in a divorce due to the severe depression plaguing the friend.

Relationships and Depression

Each side has a view. This view may be in line with the other side or it might be completely different, and

somewhere in the middle is the truth to everything.
Depression and relationships are like this.

You are in a dark place. Everything you see around
you is negative. The things that should be bringing
you happiness are not. You also feel that no one can
understand. You tend to withdraw. There is also a
high likelihood that you are complaining about many
things to yourself and to your friends. Every little
thing can be a complaint, when depression has its
hooks in you.

The deep relationships you have are often able to deal
with this side of you. Their love demands that they
help you work through the troubles, at least for a time.
Those who love you want the best, they want to be
able to fix your problems, but their own problems can
start to stack up. They can begin to affect the person,
so they are unable to help you.

If it gets to be too much or you are too unwilling to
seek help, then the loved one may pull away. They
may try to seek happiness elsewhere or simply give up
on you. The strength that exists in your relationship
will determine whether a person is willing to stay by
your side, through the tough times and provide the
care you need.

Some relationships are not strong enough. Sometimes
divorce or avoidance is the only way your loved one
can handle the depressive state you are in. People

tend to seek happiness, when surrounded by unhappiness. They don't want to feel as sad and depressed as you. If they struggle with their own depression, then they may also pull away.

Since depression often means sleeping a lot, stopping the hobbies you used to love, and having a lack of concentration, relationships are often the first to be harmed. A person with depression may refuse to do anything that used to be enjoyable, leaving the one in the relationship without depression to wonder why the person is pulling away. It is a cycle that can injure relationships forever.

The one truth is that the person you love does not want to pull away. They do not want to seek a different relationship, but at some point they are going to realize that they are either enabling your depressive state or they are unable to help you because it is hurting them.

A caregiver, even one that loves you and is there for you, has to take care of themselves and their needs before they can help you.

Health

Relationships are not the only area of your life to suffer. Medically, your mind is a powerful tool capable of many things, including making you sick. Depression may be a manifestation of your negative emotions, but it can be expressed in severe, chronic pain.

If there is no underlying health condition causing your depression like thyroid disorder, you can make your back, head, or your entire body ache. You can make yourself feel ill, as if you have some horrible disease, and yet have depression. This pain makes you want to ignore the fun things you use to do in life. You might even wish to lay in bed all day because of the pain and yet, this will not provide a release of the pain.

Depression can also bring on IBS symptoms. Perhaps irritable bowel syndrome is actually more prevalent because of the high rate of depression. This is unknown, but one thing is for certain—when you suffer from depression your insides suffer.

People with depression have reported IBS with diarrhea. Their stomach becomes so upset, it gets nauseous, and requires many bathroom trips. Each time you have this issue, you are hurting your body even more. You can start developing ulcers and hemorrhoids.

Work

Work is greatly affected, whether you show up or not. First, if you do go to work or speak with co-workers when you telecommute, you are often negative. You also tend to avoid doing your job. If you have deadlines, you start missing these deadlines. The quality of your work suffers, and eventually, you are seen as not performing your duties correctly. This can lead to you losing your job.

If you admit to the depression, then you have an out, but only for a short time. Your boss or bosses will only care for a short time that you have a problem. They will still want to see you returning to a proper performance level.

Depression can also be a hindrance for you going to work at all. There are times when a person with depression calls in sick or requests more time off than they are paid for. These constant call-ins usually lead to attendance issues, and companies tend to have a policy of "excessive" call-ins. You can be put on notice that one more missed day in a certain time period will be the end of your job.

Chapter 6: Techniques to Boost Your Self-Esteem

Self-esteem is one area that is greatly affected by depression. It can also be a cause of depression. There are techniques you can use to boost your self-esteem. These techniques do not work for everyone with depression as it does have a lot to do with the level of severity. However, working on these techniques can start to help you in numerous ways. Setbacks are okay; it is when you give up that you are hurting yourself and others.

1. Positive self-talk is the hardest thing for someone with depression. A journal can be a helpful tool. Each morning or every night before bed, write down one positive aspect of your day or about yourself. Even one positive thought can help you change what you are feeling. It may not last more than 10 minutes, but the fact that you are retraining your brain to focus on the positive for a short time, will start to become a routine.

   A routine got you into the negative thinking you do, so a new routine of positive thoughts for a short time can get you out of it. Positive talk about yourself is also a way to feel good about who you are.

2. You should not compare yourself to someone else. It can be hard. You have all these people around you and they seem to have a "perfect" world. The trouble is, you are often misled into thinking their world is perfect. Like you, people hide the true nature of their life. It is possible for someone to be depressed, even more depressed than you and not show it.

Another person might have many money worries and constantly be fighting with their spouse before a divorce happens suddenly. Comparing yourself to another is going to make you feel bad about yourself, and a lot of what you see isn't the reality.

3. Perfection is something you must let go. You cannot reach perfection because the world is not perfect. Is a mountain perfect? Is a tree? No. Even a symmetrical building can have something that is slightly off. As the human race, no one is perfect no matter how much we try. By continuing to try, you are hurting yourself. Let the control fall away and live life.

4. Exercise is known to release happy endorphins. These endorphins help you feel good about yourself because you are doing something to

improve yourself. When self-esteem and depression are combined, it is very difficult for you to choose to exercise.

It takes a lot of drive, even if you pay to use a fitness center. But, every time you exercise you are going to feel energized, better about yourself, and have the endorphins to feel happy. Exercise also helps you keep your health.

5. If you make a mistake move on. Our brains tend to overanalyze mistakes. One trick that has been learned is to choose music that helps you feel peaceful. For example, ocean waves for deep sleep, is a channel on streaming radios. This channel offers various soft piano music and ocean wave sounds. Sometimes there are also birds chirping.

These sounds can help your body and mind relax, giving you the opportunity to tell your brain you are not going to think about the mistakes you made for the day. A lot of building your self-esteem and ending your depression is in telling yourself you are not "going to dwell on the bad," and will think of a positive thought.

6. Self-esteem requires that you start doing things you enjoy. Depression stops you from doing

what you enjoy, and yet the solution to both depression and self-esteem is to get back into your hobbies. If you need to have a friend help you with this. You might be hesitant to go out, but the right friend will push you to.

7. Always give yourself a reward, even for the small accomplishments you have done. For example, if you have written 10,000 words in a book, celebrate it. It might not be the whole book, but at least you reached a milestone.

8. Start focusing on the things you can change about yourself or the situation you are in. If you feel down because of money, go back to school, get a second job, or change careers.

Increasing your self-esteem will take time. Depression can get in the way of progress, but accept that, move on from it, and keep plugging away at changing yourself and soon depression may start to correct itself.

Chapter 7: Treatment for Depression

Treatment for depression comes in many forms. One of these treatment forms may be suitable for you. However, know that researchers are also working on new approaches to treating depression that may be better suited for you.

Drugs

Medications are a temporary cure for depression. Medications are something you can build a intolerance to. They can also cause more depression in you, depending on your body and mind.

Some individuals who have taken anti-depressants actually feel more fatigue and suicidal. Citalopram is a common anti-depressant given for depression. Reports indicate that 30% of people on this medication find they are used to it within a few months and their symptoms are no longer being taken care of. Medications can also lead to addictions and health issues. Most anti-depressants have a long list of side effects, do's and don'ts that are not good for you.

Therapy

Numerous types of therapy exist. Cognitive behavior therapy (CBT) is the most common therapy used by psychologists today. It has been effective for many people, but there are also setbacks with this type of therapy. CBT requires you to actively attempt to retrain the way you think.

In therapy and on your own, you are asked to record your negative thought. What was the situation that caused this negative thought? How did you react? What are five or more ways, you could have reacted better? The idea is that if you face the same situation again, you are able to think of a more positive response and use it. It is also a therapy, where you are asked to slow down and assess the situation.

If you stop, think, listen, correct your internal reaction, then you are able to gain a better overall reaction in various situations. Let's assess an example.

Say you are at work. You made a mistake. You are in a depressive state. You call yourself stupid, you say it aloud to others, and you are unhappy the rest of the day.

In therapy, you would be asked to stop, think about those thoughts, and listen to how harmful they are.

You would then need to determine how you could have reacted better, such as saying "I made a mistake. It does not make me less of a person, but I do need to learn from this mistake, and try to avoid it in the future."

In this way, you acknowledge the problem, you accept that mistakes happen because people are not perfect, and you will learn from it in the future.

Therapy can also be one-on-one sessions, where you talk about your feelings. Sometimes you just need to talk, to unload, and you are able to see things clearly. It is not complaining or useless time, as long as the person helping you works with depression. You want someone who is an expert in depression versus a common therapist or counselor, particularly if you have severe depression.

Support Groups

Support groups should be used in conjunction with therapy. Support groups provide you with a place to go and talk about your troubles, with others who share the same troubles. Seeing that others are in difficult situations and depressed can help you reflect on your own behavior.

Changing Relationships

Not all relationships are healthy for you. Some relationships enable you to continue being depressed. Other relationships are not giving you what you need, such as support and attention. Changing these relationships can help you find your self-worth and get on the path to recovery.

Herbal Remedies

St. John's Wart is just one herb known to help with depression on a short-term basis. There are also teas with herbs in them that are known to help with depression because they help calm you and correct hormonal imbalances. Herbs are not always the answer and should not be taken unless you speak with a physician or mental health professional first.

Chapter 8: New Approaches and Methods to Treat Depression

Researchers are consistently looking for ways to treat depression. There is not a specific cure all for depression. Some treatments work for certain patients, but not to others. To a degree, researchers are still asking questions about why depression occurs. Yes, there are certainly specific causes depression has been linked to; however, there some individuals that find no help in current treatments.

There are still unanswered questions about the hereditary properties of depression in certain family groups. All of these unanswered questions are leading researchers towards new methods of treatment, with the aim of treating more patients successfully.

One new approach to depression has targeted brain dysfunctions, cognitive, and emotional processes, which trigger depression symptoms. Greg J. Siegle is the director of the Program in Cognitive Affective Neuroscience, located at the University of Pittsburgh School of Medicine. Dr. Siegle states their new approach is to think of the brain as a muscle, which has atrophied, like the heart muscle atrophies during a stroke. He believes the brain is a muscle that needs to be rehabbed.

Their efforts have been to study the effects of computer games, math problems, and audio chirping birds to stimulate the emotional regulation of the brain. Other researchers use words and faces to help depressed individuals to disengage from the negative stimuli and focus on positive stimuli.

Computer games are used along with electrical stimulation of the brain in some studies. These treatments have mixed results. Scientists are working to determine the appropriate doses and they know that this therapy protocol will not work for all patients. The concept behind the new approach is to try something for individuals that have certain brain dysfunction leading to depression.

Scientists have taken images of depressed brains to try to map the areas of the brain affected by the disorder. They are working on treatments that target these areas in an attempt to "heal" the brain (Petersen, 2015).

Cognitive Control Training

Dr. Siegle is just one of the professionals working on depression treatments, who believe old therapies are not offering the greatest help possible. Simon Rego is the director of psychology training located at the Montefiore Medical Center in New York. Dr. Rego believes cognitive behavioral therapy or CBT is too hard for people suffering from depression. CBT is a retraining of the brain to stop thinking negatively, by analyzing the situation, your reaction, and coming up with positive ways to assess the emotions.

Dr. Rego feels people who are depressed have low energy, motivation, and concentration. It is difficult for a therapy to ask for a task to be completed that is opposite of what one's energy level is.

CCT is his alternative suggestion. With Cognitive Control Training, a person suffering from depression is asked to perform two exercises that last 15 minutes each. The patients are given numbers that are in a series. These numbers have set rules. The task is an attempt to activate an area of the prefrontal cortex called the dorsal lateral. It is the part of the brain associated with emotion regulation, as well as executive control. Dr. Siegle states it is an area that "voluntarily thinks" about something when you want it to. Dr. Siegle is part of the team that has developed CCT. He believes this underactive area of the brain is why many people ruminate on negative thoughts, which plague them, and make them feel depressed.

CCT includes listening to the sounds of birds chirping. These external sounds culminated with active and direct attention on the sounds, allows a person to concentrate on something other than their own thoughts.

The report, published in Behavioral and Cognitive Psychotherapy discussed a study that involved 48 people. These people suffered from depression. They were given three sessions of CCT. These sessions occurred in a two-week period. The depression scores dropped more significantly, than people obtaining CBT control exercises. The study was published in 2014.

A group located in Australia has also examined CCT with trans cranial direct current stimulation (tDCS). An electric current, on a gentle setting, is used while video games are played. A study called Brain Stimulation was published in 2014 based on this study. It showed depressed patients who had a combination of CCT and electrical stimulation experienced a 46% reduction in their symptoms after three weeks of treatment. Individuals who received only CCT saw a decrease in symptoms of only 17% and those with electrical stimulation only saw an 8.9% reduction.

Among the new therapies developed, Dr. Siegle has worked on exercises in concentration. He uses two electrodes on the arm, passing a very weak current through the body. The placement of the electrode causes an itching sensation that is extremely annoying. Patients find it difficult to think negative thoughts with this itching occurring (Petersen, 2015).

Interpretation Bias Modification

Interpretation Bias Modification is also called Cognitive Bias Modification-Interpretation (CBM-I). It is a new treatment Dr. Jamie Micco, at Harvard Medical School has been working on. Micco is an assistant professor. He stated CBM-I tries to contradict the way people look at ambiguous situations and then react negatively.

In one study, he had patients look at written scenarios. These scenarios were positively resolved, but often the last word was missing a letter and patients needed to fill it in. CBM-I's goal is to help patients think in a positive or neutral way, versus the negative their brain's focus on.

Further testing for CBM-I treatment has people look at two faces, one neutral in expression and the other sad. The patient is trained to look away from the negative and focus on the neutral, just as the patient is asked to focus on neutral words versus negative words.

The Journal of Abnormal Psychology published a study in 2015 relating to CBM as a way to reduce negative focus. The treatment contained a placebo, where 52 subjects were studied for four weeks. Patients noticed a 40% reduction in symptoms. The study's authors thought the placebo treatment actually enhanced the attention of patients, which helped reduce the symptoms patients felt.

The new approaches discussed focus mainly on the negative attention depressed patients have. They are biased towards negative thoughts versus positive thoughts. About 2/3 thirds of patients with depression have these rumination troubles, and the other third do not. It is very important for a trained professional to treat a patient with depression based on their symptoms, reactions to situations, and physical well-being. To be successful one has to understand the neurobiological and cognitive issue in the patient, so that treatment can be designed specifically for the patient (Petersen, 2015).

Treatment-Resistant Depression Approaches

Neuromodulation is one type of treatment patients are incorporating into their depression treatment, when all other methods have failed. It is designed to pass electrical current through the brain.

There are a couple of types of this treatment: electroconvulsive therapy, Vagus nerve stimulation and repetitive transcranial magnetic stimulation. These all use a type of weak electrical current that is transmitted by the electrodes. They work on stimulating specific areas of the brain, such as the Vagus nerve (University of Michigan, 2016).

The Vagus nerve supplies the lungs, heart, upper digestive tract and other organs. It is a cranial nerve that provides parasympathetic control of these organs. Research studies indicate stimulating these organs and the nerve can relieve pain, but also help a person retrain their brain to think in a more positive manner. It is also a nerve that Psychology Today links with "gut instincts."

A study in Switzerland found the nerve provides feelings, what we call gut instincts to the brain. These are the instinctual feelings that tell us when there is danger or when we have the right answer. By using electrical current, the nerve is stimulated to feel less "threatening" feelings, thus allowing happier thoughts to enter the brain.

This and the other treatments discussed are in early testing. Only small groups of people have been tested. As new approaches, these treatments are seemingly positive for certain types of patients.

If you have tried other treatments, without success or feel that CBT is too much work for your current depressive state, you may wish to find a study near you or ask your current physician/therapist about these options.

The more information you gather about potential help with your depression, the more comfortable and in control you will start to feel. Depending on the severity of your depression, a small step of gaining control can push you towards a more energetic reaction. It could provide you with the desire needed to get your brain engaged, actively, in treating your depression versus losing interest or concentration again and again.

When one therapy does not work, do not give up. You just have not found the right therapy for you. It does exist, but it also takes work and the driving need to want the help.

Chapter 9: Who Can Help You Most

Treatment for depression is like any other disease—you have to want to receive help, in order to get better. You are the person who can help you the most, when it comes to your depression.

Admitting Something is Wrong

It is difficult to admit when something does not feel right. It is even more difficult if you have lived in a cycle for years, without noticing when it started. If you feel you have depression and picked up this book, then you have taken the first step in admitting something is wrong.

For those who are looking to help their loved ones, it is not impossible, but they have to want the help. You might try a few of these suggestions:

- "Wow that was a really negative response, I've noticed more pessimism in your responses lately, is there anything you feel is bothering you?" This type of statement points out you noticed, you care, and you are not labeling their "negativity. Instead, you are asking if you can help alleviate a "regular" concern.

- Try leaving out materials about depression. Sometimes a person knows they need help, but is unwilling to ask for it. Providing the materials that give them a helpline may allow the person to admit something is wrong.

- Fiction can be another way of pointing out situations to a loved one. Watch a show with a character battling depression. Make comments about the show, they should be positive and insightful, but point out some of the behavior or the reactions the character has. Often times people see things in others before they are willing to see it in themselves.

- You can also plan a visit for a regular physical for the loved one. This is more difficult in older individuals, but it can still be accomplished. It may not work because the person has to be willing to answer the questions on the intake form correctly.

- However, if you are able to be in the room, you can also voice your concerns. These concerns don't have to include the word "depression," just a statement of "casual" observations, such as "you seem more tired recently" or "I have not seen you enjoying x hobby." It gives the doctor a way to ask questions about depression, without you pointing the finger that you have them all diagnosed.

Changing your Situation

Once there is an admittance of an issue, it is time to look for ways to change your situation. It may not be within you that changes need to be made in this step. For example, a young woman with thyroid troubles faced depression. However, taking her medication regularly was not helping with the imbalances she was feeling in her own body.

As an observant individual, she tracked her outburst and depression to the two weeks and sometimes a week before her menstrual cycle started. She was exhibiting earlier signs of PMS than usual, as well as more drastic anger, depression, and emotions during the PMS phase.

This young woman spoke with her physician about these symptoms, but received no reply. Taking it upon herself, she researched information about depression, changes in hormones, and couldn't find any concrete proof that reaching over 30 years of age may cause a change in her menstrual cycle.

However, it was clearly happening. Again, going to the physician she asked if, other than her thyroid troubles, something might have changed with her hormones. Again, the physician did not provide a proper reply. Armed with information that St. John's Wart, when used in limited quantities, could help with depression, she asked if she could start taking it. The idea was to take the herbal medicine a week or two prior to her period start date and see if there was an improvement.

After four months, she discovered a significant improvement. Taking a pill on a daily basis for a week prior to her period, this young woman had an easier time during the PMS stage. Her body also returned to normal, with fewer depressive episodes and she was able to track that every other month she suffered from worse PMS symptoms, with significant depression.

You may have to take the initiative in your health care and mental care. While physicians should be relied on for their expert medical knowledge, you may have to change how you approach your own care.

The example is not about the woman seeking her own medical advice online, but about reading information, so she was better armed to speak with her physician about her symptoms.

It is also about what else you can change. Feeling depressed, dealing with a busy life, and money concerns, she was unable to take action to find a new physician that might have heard her concerns with a better "bedside manner."

The experience has taught this person that if the physician is not going to learn, then it is paramount to her overall well-being to seek a new general practitioner. Your care is in your hands. You ultimately decide if you are going to follow a care plan, but you also have to have a physician who is willing to listen, take you seriously, and see your intelligence.

Depression is all about feeling unintelligent and worthless. You don't need a physician who is not going to listen or search for the underlying cause of your feelings. Rather, you need a person who will listen, who will refer you to the right people, and the person who is willing to help you.

You are the most important person in your care plan. You are the person who has to make changes to your situation to alleviate the turmoil you feel. When you are ready to accept these needs, you are ready to find a treatment plan that will work for you. Only when you are ready to seek help are you truly going to get the help you need. It comes from within you, as well as from the resources you have at your disposal.

Chapter 10: How to Find Fulfillment in Life

You can begin your own treatment. If you have sought a diagnosis from a physician or psychologist, you can work towards a treatment plan with them, as well as with yourself. Depression has many causes, but among them and often the most prevalent is feeling worthless, stupid, and low self-esteem. This cycle of emotions can be broken. These steps may not work for everyone. You may have tried them and found no success, but perhaps it was your self-discipline and approach.

The Mind is a Powerful Organ

Your mind is extremely powerful. It is the epicenter of your entire life. Without your brain, you would be an empty shell. The phrase "you cannot teach an old dog new tricks," is a myth. Worse, it is wrong. You can teach your aging brain new tricks. You can change how it reacts, thinks, and processes information. All you need to do is be willing and discover any underlying factors that might hinder this process.

Here are some things that may make these steps difficult:

- You have an illness, you do not know about, thyroid disorder, beginnings of dementia, or other hormonal imbalance.

- You suffer from a chemical imbalance.

- Your brain may not be connected properly via the nervous system.

- Genetic causes might be affecting your brain process.

- You are in the middle of a great loss, which is making your depression worse.

- You have PTSD (post-traumatic stress disorder) that is leading to depression.

Make absolutely certain that your depression is not a result of a biological condition. Also, assess the rest of your life to determine if PTSD, abuse, or a death in your immediate family/friends circle is making your depression worse. Armed with the best list of causes for your depression, means you are armed to correct all aspects of the depression, as well as gain fulfillment from life.

Your Treatment Plan

Beginning with the understanding of your depressions cause, you can now work on a self-treatment plan to find joy in life.

1. Get a journal or start one on your computer.

2. Keep this journal with you at all times.

3. On the first page, write out 1 positive feeling about yourself. It may be that you love your hair color, its length, or your eyes. You might write that you love the strength you have in difficult situations. No matter what it is, it needs to be a compliment.

4. Underneath this compliment, write 1 goal for your life. This goal can be obtaining a new job, going back to school, finishing school, travelling somewhere. The only caveat is the goal has to be something you can accomplish, realistically.

5. If it is a goal, such as going back to school, then your job is to take small steps towards this

long term goal. It can also be a short term goal. You might set a goal about waking up, lying in bed for 10 minutes, and thinking only of positive thoughts. Whatever goal you set, you need to be able to make it.

6. The next task is to create a meaning of life chart, diagram, map, or list. This is not about goals. It is about what would make life more meaningful to you. The Buddhists believe that the end to suffering is to forgo the materialistic things and desires we have. If you desire love and you have been unable to attain it, then you may feel depressed. So what are the things that have greater meaning?

How to see the Greater Meaning

When in the throes of depression, it is difficult, nearly impossible to see the greater meaning to your life. You tend to feel worthless versus meaningful. However, all is not lost.

Writing out your emotions is the best way to find what is most meaningful to you. A person lost her father. Her father was a friend and a mentor, as well as a loved one.

Instead, of being sad and angry at the loss, she focused on the meaning he gave to her life, the happy moments that they shared together. She did not forget about the times when they argued when she was growing up, but instead, remembered the lessons from those times.

She also had the most important lesson he gave to her and that was, "I have lived my life with no regrets." Her father taught her that all mistakes, disappointments, and happiness in life is where the meaning of life comes from. It is not about dwelling on the bad, on the things that cannot be changed, but the focus should be on the positive that was gained from any situation.

Those words held more power in getting over her depression and sense of loss than any others. Perhaps they can for you as well. Take time now to consider what has happened in your life that was good.

Was there a time you felt worthwhile? Was there a person who made you feel worthy and important? If you can find one happy memory, then you can start to recall the others. From this, you can discover true meaning in your life.

Most of us do not want to feel like our existence is for naught. Yet, we also know that life ends. You are born, you live, and you die. In death, the only thing that could bring meaning to your life is how you are remembered. For some, it is about accomplishing great feats—perhaps writing the great American novel. For others, it is the family they have, the lessons they have left behind, and the community influence they have provided.

You are not going to find the meaning in your life immediately. It can take a week, a month, a year, or several years. The point is not rushing to a solution about your depression and finding fulfillment immediately, but about the trip it takes you to get there. It is also about the changes you make, so you can get to a point of realizing what fulfillment truly means.

Conclusion

Thank you again for purchasing this book!

I hope this book was able to help you with your needs and to satisfy your reading pleasures.

Depression might have been misunderstood in the beginning, and we may not fully understand the disorder now. However, we are gaining more ground in our research around the world to start helping us find better treatment opportunities.

There is a cure for you. It may be a long road, with setbacks. If you are willing to take a journey to find more meaning in your life, then you will start to find a treatment plan that fits your needs.

You do have to admit to needing help, seek a professional who can help you, and you will start to feel better about yourself. Take the next step and start feeling better.

Finally, if you enjoyed this book, please take the time to share your thoughts and post a review on Amazon. It would be greatly appreciated!

Thank you and good luck!

References

Hall, A. (2014, September 03). *10 Depression Myths We need to Stop Believing*. Retrieved from Huffington Post: http://www.huffingtonpost.com/2014/09/03/depression-myths_n_5715453.html

Medicine Net. (n.d.). *Causes of Depression*. Retrieved from Medicine Net: http://www.medicinenet.com/script/main/art.asp?articlekey=55167

Petersen, A. (2015, June 1). *To Treat Depression, a new Approach Tries Training the Brain*. Retrieved from WSJ: http://www.wsj.com/articles/to-treat-depression-a-new-approach-tries-training-the-brain-1433178996

Reiss, N. (2007, September 19). *Historical Understandings of Depression*. Retrieved from Mental Help: https://www.mentalhelp.net/articles/historical-understandings-of-depression/

University of Michigan. (2016). *Three Minute Tips New Approaches for Treating Depression*. Retrieved from Psych Med U of Michigan: http://www.psych.med.umich.edu/expert-advice/treating-depression/

Webmd. (n.d.). *Depression Health Center*. Retrieved from Web MD: http://www.webmd.com/depression/guide/detecting-depression

Wikipedia. (2016, May 27). *History of Depression.* Retrieved from Wikipedia: https://en.wikipedia.org/wiki/History_of_dep ression#20th_and_21st_centuries

World Health Organization. (2016, April). *Depression Fact Sheet.* Retrieved from WHO: http://www.who.int/mediacentre/factsheets/fs 369/en/

Charisma: Unshackle your True Charismatic Self and Improve your Social and People Skills

Be a More Confident, Charming, and Charismatic Person

By Sammy Parker

Table of Contents

Conclusion

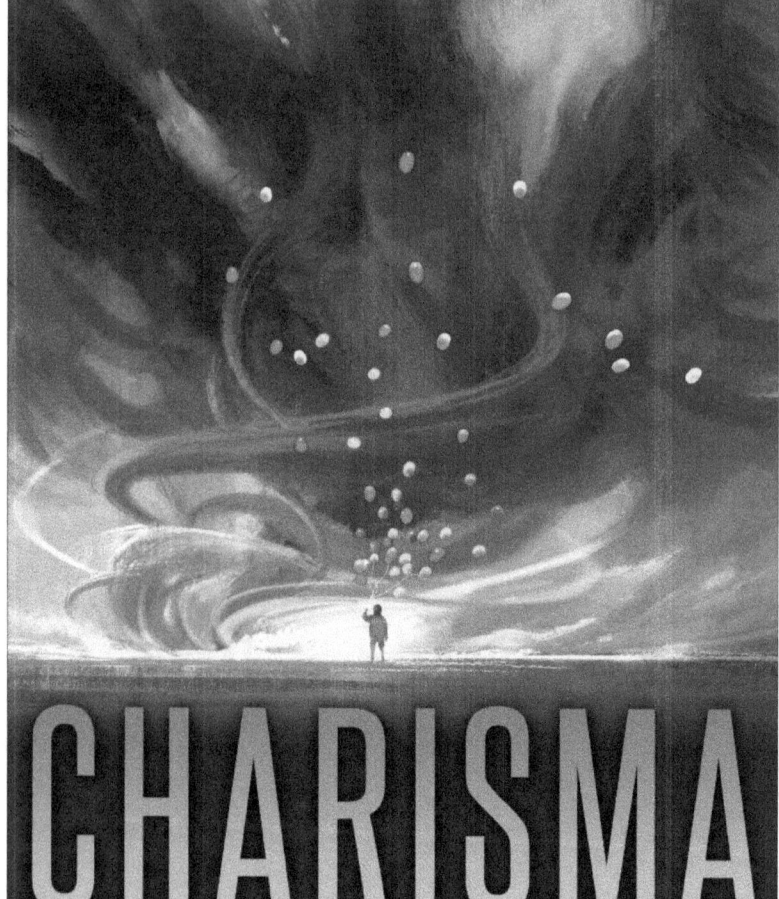

CHARISMA

UNSHACKLE YOUR TRUE CHARISMATIC SELF AND IMPROVE YOUR SOCIAL AND PEOPLE SKILLS

Be A More Confident, Charming, and Charismatic Person

SAMMY PARKER

Introduction: What is Charisma?

I want to thank you and congratulate you for downloading the book, *"Charisma"*.

This book contains proven steps and strategies on how to define what charisma means for you, personally, discover what specific factors are holding you back from achieving it in your life, and becoming a more confident and charismatic person. This book has been written with the intention to help anyone improve their charisma levels, no matter who they are. So what, exactly, does this magic word mean?

What Qualities make a Person Charismatic?

Charisma refers to your ability to influence, charm, and appeal to those you are surrounded with. This quality is often described as something that is inexplicable and mysterious, something you either have or don't have. However, it's easier than you may believe to determine what qualities make a person a charismatic individual. Some of these qualities are optimism, exuberance, confidence, a habit of smiling a lot, active body language, and more.

What does Science have to say about Charisma?

In addition to confidence and a smiley persona, studies suggest that the quality of charisma has a lot to do with the ability to think quickly. Research from a journal called Psychological Science has shown that individuals who had an easier time responding fast to visual tests or questions pertaining to general information were perceived, by others, as having higher charisma. This shows that being socially intelligent has to do with more than simply saying the right thing or acting the right way. You must be able to follow through on actions, and how well one can do this has a lot to do with how quickly their minds function.

Mental Quickness Plays a Large Role in this Quality:

Since charisma is often considered a quality in a person that is hard to define or pinpoint reasons for, this has led researchers to try to determine exactly what it is that makes some people more charismatic than others. They have found that being quick in reaction time is directly related to how charismatic one appears to others. This could be because it helps with the ability to recover quickly from awkward situations or think up clever jokes on the spot.

Anyone can Learn to become More Charismatic:

The good news is that it's a myth that you are either born with charisma or not. Anyone can develop this quality, become more confident, get better at impressing others and winning friends, and succeeding in life, in general. In this book, you will receive a THOROUGH guide that will give you a huge head start on your journey to self-fulfillment and achievement.

Thanks again for downloading this book, I hope you enjoy it!

Chapter 1: Why is Charisma Important?

If you make it a point to ask around, you will find that defining charisma is not an easy task for most people, especially in relation to social norms or communication. What it comes down to is that charisma comes from being adept with skills on an interpersonal level. The great news is, these skills can not only be learned at any age, but can also be *constantly* developed and improved. When you look at it in its most basic way, charisma is having an ability to bring good feelings to other people just by being present. A huge portion of what this means is knowing how to make others feel important. Charismatic people know how to make whomever is speaking feel truly listened to.

This may lead you to wonder how it's possible to make others feel like this. A great place to begin is by focusing your attention on a person's most positive attributes. While many people interact with others in hopes of showcasing how funny or cool they are, charismatic people like to show people that the person they are talking to is interesting. This leads people to start feeling good around the charismatic person and hoping to spend more and more time with them. Needless to say, this quality is helpful in many areas.

What Opportunities does Charisma Lead to?

- **Career Advancement:** People cannot help but respect and admire someone who has a lot of charisma. This means that you will have an easier time advancing in your career, whatever it may be. Whether you work under a boss or have hopes of running your own office someday, having a charismatic personality will aid you along the way and increase your chances for success.

- **A Better Understanding of Humanity:** Having a lot of friends and having people open up to you on a regular basis means that you will gain a better understanding of what social structures are all about. You will learn, on average, what people like and dislike, the best ways to make friends, mistakes to avoid, and more. In essence, you can view all of your interactions with humans as practice and a way to gain a better understanding of humanity as a whole. This will make you an all-around smarter person.

- **Better Luck with Love:** Being charismatic means becoming appealing to attractive people who you never would have dreamed of approaching before. Since being charismatic has to do with making others feel special and important, this works very well for attracting a mate or even casual dating. You may find that you struggled to find dates before and, after developing charisma, have to choose between different options for what to do with your Friday night.

- **More Trust from Others:** People can't help but trust a charismatic person because of the positive vibe they bring. More trust means gaining friends easier, having better luck in love, more responsibilities and chances for advancement at work, and more. Trust is an integral part of what it means to function as a social being in our society. If you can't gain the trust of others, you won't go far. For this reason, learning how to be charismatic (and, as a consequence, trustworthy) is a must for everyone.

Now that we've gone over some of the reasons why charisma is such an important ingredient in any well-rounded personality, we can get down to the best ways to go about acquiring it.

How can you be More Charismatic in Everyday Life?

Making it a point to become a more charismatic person has to do with being aware of the way you interact with those around you, since the qualities that determine how much charisma you have appeal to other people and are perceived as positive attributes. Someone with charisma knows how to use their abilities to get others to side with them. This could apply to social situations, ideological positions, or even job-related or professional concerns or situations. Because of this, charisma often has a strong association in people's minds with general leadership, which has a lot to do with how much charisma an individual has.

In order to be influential, you have to be liked by others, and in order to be liked, charisma is absolutely necessary. This is why leadership is closely related to charismatic traits. If you ask the average person to call to mind someone that has a strongly charismatic personality, their first thought will probably be a celebrity, leader, or politician. These examples are successful, often directly because of how charismatic they are, but this trait is not only reserved for the famous or well-known names out there. A lot of normal people possess high levels of charisma, as well, such as the waitress who always gets tipped the highest, the nice person at work who is friends with everyone, or the popular kids in the class.

What Separates Charismatic People from Non-charismatic People?

It's very true, in an undeniable way, that charisma is not something that everyone has equal amounts of. Some people draw in and captivate lots of people, while others only seem to do so every once in a while or even, in extreme cases, repel people. Charisma is magnetic to everyone. It can be very easy to recognize this type of personality, but harder to sum up what it is about their personality that is so magnetic.

What does being Charismatic Refer to?

- **Having Healthy Confidence:** People who are considered charismatic are also considered confident. This can mean that they either are genuinely confident, or know how to appear that way to others. Having the confidence to communicate with others in many different situations, whether it be in front of people, in small groups, or one on one chats, is a quality that does not come easily to everyone. In fact, this is something that a lot of people struggle with.

Someone who has charisma does not only look confident as they communicate with others, but also helps other people feel more confident in themselves, which enhances and aides the process of communication, in general. They know how to get people excited and involved with the subject matter at hand and often have a positive effect on those they interact with in life. They have a healthy type of confidence that never comes off as arrogant or boastful.

- **They Look on the Bright Side:** Similar to being or appearing confident, charismatic people are often very optimistic, or at least know how to look that way to others. They will always look for the best in events, situations, or those around them, no matter what. Their peace of mind does not depend on everything around them going perfectly, but instead comes from a calm knowing that things have a tendency to work out.

People with this magical quality know how to encourage people to view situations the same way as them, meaning that they can influence others to become more positive and optimistic, about specific scenarios as well as in general. Both optimism and general positivity are important forces for solving problems or negotiating successfully with other people, both in professional and personal situations.

- **They Know how to Keep their Emotions in Check:** A charismatic person does not become outwardly frazzled or overreact to simple issues. They know how to keep the appearance of being optimistic and confident even if that isn't what they are feeling inside at the time. They also know that it's important not to let emotions take over and cloud judgment in any situations.

It's true that people with charisma are great at revealing their truest feelings when it works in their favor, but they tend to also be good at maintaining composure in any situation, even if on the inside they are not feeling very calm or confident.

- **Being Interested in Other People as well as Interesting:** People who have charisma interactions on an interpersonal level. It has to do with knowing how to communicate with others in a dynamic way, with plenty of enthusiasm and passion, always using body language in a positive and energizing way. This has to do with being an optimistic person who has a lot of self-confidence, and knowing how to gain the trust and respect of those around you.

Now that you are aware of some of the traits that go hand in hand with being charismatic, you can start to observe whether or not they are present in your own life and start thinking of ways to develop these qualities. Everyone can learn to become more charismatic, getting stronger in interpersonal communication with knowledge and plenty of practice. Remember that although charismatic people may be very well liked, on average, it isn't possible to please everyone and that should never be your goal.

confidence in them.

- **Knowing how to Act Assertive:** One of the great powers of this personality trait is being able to come together for a common reason or to believe in what you wish for them to believe in. Obviously, a skill like this can be used for good causes or bad ones. Leaders with charisma are able to encourage and influence the people who follow them, knowing exactly how to motivate others for specific purposes. Tricksters with high levels of charisma and confidence will likely be able to use their qualities quite easily to get the respect and trust of people before taking advantage of them in some way.

People with charisma have plenty of assertiveness, but in a way that is quite subtle. They are able to persuade others using speech, motivate and encourage other people with confidence and positivity, and use assertiveness by making use of their knowledge of their own feelings and the feelings of other people.

- **Knowing how to Focus on Detail that Others may not Notice:** Being charismatic has a lot to do with knowing which details to pay attention to, especially when it comes to

A charismatic individual is never too self-absorbed to be interested in what another person has to say, and it shows. This means that they will typically ask questions in an open way with the intention of getting a better understanding of the speaker and their feelings or opinions. Due to their skill for making other people feel comfortable, they will often receive real and honest answers from others. A person with charisma tends to be considerate and empathetic with other people, taking the time to recall details about individuals from previous meetings, which does a lot to build rapport and respect.

- **Showing your own Intelligence to Others:** Charismatic people hope to communicate in effective ways with people around them, meaning that they usually know how to start conversations with other people. On average, they are quite smart with a general knowledge of topics that makes connecting with many different personality types possible.

They also tend to have expertise in one specific area, along with the ability to tell others about it in an understandable and digestible way. This involves being able to adapt what they are saying to the knowledge of the person they are speaking with. This type of expertise and knowledge will make others have more are very interesting people to those around them, meaning that people enjoy listening to them and are curious about the details of their lives. This goes hand in hand with the fact that they are also interested in those around them, taking the time to stop and listen thoroughly when another is speaking to them.

People with charisma are oftentimes great at telling stories, adopting an energetic vibe when they explain ideas or speak their thoughts or memories. This makes them able to get messages across in a concise and clear manner, using humor when appropriate and being serious at other times. They know how to perfectly balance the two as to keep listeners engaged with what they are saying.

- **Knowing how to Adopt Inviting Body Language:** When these people are in smaller groups or one on one conversation, they will often have a relaxed and open body language posture, complete with plenty of direct eye contact. They will stay open and aware of the reactions and moods of others, adjusting their speaking manner accordingly, if necessary. When they are in bigger groups of people or performing in some way for an audience, they will adjust their body language to be larger, with the intention of addressing a lot of people at once.

Chapter 2: Overcoming Shyness and Becoming more Confident

Many of us are afflicted with shyness. This can be something that occurs when we are children and then goes away with time, or a lifelong battle. Some people are only shy with members of the opposite sex, while others are only shy around strangers. You may start out as a shy kid and then eventually find that these shy reactions dissipate with time and you eventually become very confident in social situations. Some may believe that this is the direct result of getting older. Getting older certainly does have to do with becoming more confident since you are able to reflect on your life and see the situations that you handled well and believe in yourself more as a consequence, but that is far from the entire picture.

What Causes so Many People to Suffer from a Lack of Confidence?

Everyone on this earth is, at their core, a social creature. We are built to survive and thrive in communities, engaged with other people either daily or most days of our lives. Whether this community is small or large doesn't matter. To see an example of this need for social interaction, you only need to look at the way inmates react to being put into solitary confinement. Being separated from others for an extended period of time is considered a very cruel and harsh form of punishment.

Regardless of this innate importance in our social relationships with the world around us, most of us get uncomfortable at the thought or action of interacting with other people, especially when we don't know them. Even people who seem the most confident outwardly are affected by what others think of them, and at times even influenced by it. Many people may claim that the opinions of others don't matter to them, but this would change quickly if everyone they knew suddenly turned against them.

How does Shyness Hold us Back in Life?

- **It Allows Others to take Advantage of us more Easily:** When a person is shy, they don't have an easy time speaking up about situations, even when that situation is negative for them. They would rather not "cause problems" or "make a big deal out of things" and will often avoid confrontation at all costs. This can turn out to be a highly negative fact, since other people may catch onto this and take advantage of the shy person.

- **We Miss out on Potential Friendships or Love:** When you are shy, you are afraid to approach people, even people you find interesting or attractive. Instead of walking up to them to find out if you two would get along or hit it off, you hide in the corner and say nothing. This is a great way to miss out on wonderful potential relationships that could change your life for the better.

- **It Causes a lot of Unnecessary Anxiety:** Being shy is stressful, and it causes you to worry about a lot of things that don't actually warrant so much thought and tension. Learning how to release your shyness is akin to dropping a huge backpack off of your back that has been weighing you down for years and realizing that it didn't hold anything useful all along. Sometimes, learning how to be less shy comes down to having more respect for yourself and not allowing your thoughts to run rampant and ruin things for you.

- **We don't get to Make our Own Reputation:** Since shy people often don't speak for themselves, others will make up the details on their own. For example, if a person gets invited to a party and doesn't interact with anyone else due to being shy, sitting in the corner, this could be perceived as rudeness.

A person who is too shy to display their personality to others or even correct others when they get it wrong, will have the misfortune of being labeled by other people, even when those labels are completely wrong. It's true that we all get labeled regardless of our personality type, but you can control this a lot more when you have confidence and are not shy.

The Maps we Make of the Minds around Us:

When we talk with people around us, we have a tendency to try to predict what the minds around us are thinking from moment to moment, during any given conversation. This means that we are always theorizing and imagining what they may be thinking about us, how they are responding to what we are saying, and also reacting and judging the imaginings we are having. For example, if we have reason to believe that a person nearby thinks we are attractive, we might feel good in response to this, imagining that they have quality taste. On the other hand, if we judge that someone finds us attractive and we disagree, we might feel even worse about ourselves subconsciously. We also tend to be hyperaware of the reactions of others after we put ourselves out there in some way, such as telling a joke.

Being Around People we Know vs. Strangers:

What shyness can be summed up as, then, is the fear of engaging with other people due to the worry that we will become embarrassed in front of them. This is why it's easy to feel shy about certain situations and completely confident in others. For example, being in a room of relatives who you have known your entire life makes becoming shy significantly less likely than being in a room of strangers, even though it doesn't make it impossible. This is because relatives are already familiar with the way we behave, our mannerisms, and other small details about us, and we are aware of the way they will react to it, for the most part.

This makes it so that we don't fear displaying our personalities, being expressive, or saying what we truly think, due to the embarrassment risk being quite low in comparison to other situations.

Uncertainty is Often the Cause of Shyness:

Being in a room with a lot of people you don't know, however, is a different situation. They have never had a chance to grow familiar with your mannerisms or opinions, leading you to wonder how they will perceive and receive you. There is no way to know this ahead of time. The willingness you have to risk putting yourself out there and being embarrassed will play a direct role in the level of shyness you feel around them.

It's also a Matter of What you Decide to Focus on:

Another fundamental reason that people get shy is that they are placing their attention in places that make this true. If you decide to focus on how others might perceive you and whether or not they will accept you, you run a higher risk of overanalyzing your own deeds, words, and thoughts. This can lead to a paralyzing state of being where you cannot stop analyzing yourself and judging those perceptions. However, if you can learn to shift your focus to other people, remembering to ignore whether or not they will accept us (while still remaining respectful and polite, of course), we might notice that we can breathe easier and become more at ease with ourselves around other people.

How to Change your Focus around Other People:

If you struggle with shyness, reading this will lead you to wonder how it is possible to shift your attention that way when it seems nearly impossible in so many situations.

The key is to work on developing a conscious interest in other people and what their concerns may be. It's a common fact that the more absorbed you become in something, the less you are focused on or obsessed with your self-image and the way others will perceive you. To put it another way, developing compassion for others can lead you to be less concerned about what they will think of you. This doesn't mean that you don't care about their ideas or thoughts, but that you are not controlled by them and don't fear them at all.

How being Understanding of Others Helps with Shyness:

If you try this out, you will notice that it seems impossible to have a genuine interest in and care for people in front of you while at the same time fearing what they think of you. This could point to compassion being a way to cure shyness. For some, it may be hard to envision entering a place full of people you don't know and realizing that they are all suffering in their own unique way. But it's true that everyone is struggling on their own with one thing or another. Sure, it may not be a huge deal, but everyone hides their own suffering to some degree.

However, you don't have to be aware of the details of each person's suffering or struggles to assume that they could use some compassion. Compassion has to do with caring about the happiness of others as much as we care about our own happiness. If you learn to approach strangers with this emotion, or even a basic interest in their lives, you will find that it is much harder to be shy. Not only are you shifting your focus to something outside of you, but you are willfully becoming more positive about your interactions with others and how you view them. Eventually, shyness will become less of a problem or even vanish completely without a trace. This idea supposes that getting more confident is not all about feeling better about yourself, but also caring about others.

Some Other Ways to Improve Confidence:

- **Get Involved:** When you are a part of something, whether it be a book club, sports team, or acting class, you have a chance to connect with others and less free time to engage in fears about being in adequate. Finding something to get excited about is a great way to develop a sense of self and meet like-minded people.

You can start by searching for clubs in your town on the internet and finding something that interests you, or by asking some of your friends if they are involved in activities that you could join in on. Even if it's something you would never normally partake in, you should step out of your comfort zone and do it anyway.

- **Take the Time to Look Nice:** Although confidence is something that should come from the inside, looking nice on the outside doesn't hurt. Everyone feels better about themselves when they are wearing clean clothes and have engaged in the proper hygiene for that day. Taking the time to respect your outer-appearance will go a long way in broadcasting to the world a confident person who can take on anything.

- **Start a Journal:** Part of being shy is not having awareness about ourselves well enough to feel comfortable in our own skin. We are so busy worrying about how we look and seem to others that we never take the time to get to know our own thoughts and opinions. A great way to fix this is to start a journal. Even if you aren't sure what to write at first, if you commit to one short entry a day, you will eventually discover that you are getting to know yourself much better and gradually building your confidence.

- **Approach Strangers:** This may sound unthinkable to a very shy person who doesn't enjoy interacting with strangers, but the more you do it, the easier it gets, and you will eventually wonder why you held back for so long. Every time you have an interaction with someone you don't know, there's a chance to learn something about yourself.

If you follow the steps outlined here, you will eventually notice your shyness dissipating. All of these steps work as exercises on their own or can be combined for even more effectiveness. Overcoming shyness is something that we can all improve upon. All it takes is dedication, knowledge, and practice to become better at it.

So far so good? If you don't mind, please leave an honest review of this book. I would truly appreciate it! Thank you!

Chapter 3: Anyone can Develop Charisma

There's an ongoing myth that a lot of people assume to be true, that gaining charisma is not possible and that you must be born with it. People view it as a trait that you either receive at birth or do not. However, when you look closely at charisma and the qualities that make someone charismatic, you will notice that these are all traits that can be gained and then improved over time. We have already gone over the reasons why charisma is so important in this book, so now we will review some of the ways that you can start to work on it within yourself.

Methods for Becoming a More Charismatic Person:

- **Improving your Overall Positivity:** If you have hopes to make others around you feel good, which is the essence of charisma, you have to learn how to feel good too. When someone feels upbeat and positive, this attitude comes across to others and lifts them up. When you can spread positivity in this way, you will make others feel great. Being positive isn't always easy though, so if you have a hard time getting into this mood, here's a trick you can use to improve it instantly:

Choose one of your favorite songs; a song that makes you happy any time you listen to it. This can be a song with positive associations from childhood or any song that recalls a positive memory from the past. Now, whenever you have a need to get a boost of positivity, call this song to mind and hum along with it. Dance along, move your feet, and let yourself really get into the vibe of the song. Allow the positive associations or memories attached to the song take you over and bring positivity to your mood. This will cause you to become more positive and rub off on other people around you.

- **Spread Positivity to the People around You:** Another way you can start developing your charisma is by figuring out how to spread positivity to people in your life. Learning how to be charming and positive with only certain types of people (like appealing members of the opposite sex, for example), but neglecting to relate to other people will not make you more charismatic because people will see the inconsistency in your actions. In order to avoid this trap, you must make sure you make an effort to be social and friendly to all people and not just some people.

- **Become a Giving Person:** Although being friendly and social to all people around you can help, this isn't enough. You must also learn to acquire a giving and generous and interested persona. Try searching for opportunities to make things easier or better for others instead of always trying to find out what you can receive from them.

If, for example, you approach someone with the intention of asking a favor or hoping to get them to like you, they will pick up on this and likely be unimpressed or turned off. However, if you approach people with the intention of making their day better and simply interacting with them in a fun way, this will put forth a more appealing and charismatic vibe that will draw people in.

- **Realize that it's not All about you:** We mentioned this earlier, but it's worth stating again. Being truly charismatic is not about impressing others with your greatness, but about making people feel as though they are very important and worth listening to. What this means is that you have to put forth effort to show that the people you are interacting with that you care about what they have to say.

There are a couple of ways that you can make sure this comes across in your social interactions with people. You can try this with people you know to practice and then move on to strangers to get better at it. Make a conscious effort to spend less time during conversation thinking about how you will reply to what is being said, and more time actively engaging in listening. Force yourself to refrain from interrupting, however many times you may be tempted. This will get easier with time.

You may find this difficult at first and notice that your mind wanders as you try to actively listen to others. You can bring your attention back to the conversation by zoning in on your physical body or sensations in the body. You can also try to zone in on your breath as an anchor to stay engaged and active in listening. Make sure that you also adopt a posture of listening, meaning that you are facing the person, still instead of fidgeting, and making eye contact instead of looking around. This will show that you care about what they are saying and make it so that you come across as more charismatic.

- **Connect and Open up to Other People:**
  We did just mention that it isn't all about you
  when you are talking with another person, but
  this isn't to say that you can't share your
  feelings and thoughts with the person you are
  talking to. When it comes down to it,
  conversations are a two way street with plenty
  of back and forth interaction.

  One way to make what you are saying more
  personal is to speak from an "I" perspective
  instead of a neutral or passive voice. You can
  say that you love something, rather than saying
  that something is fun. This shows that you are
  sharing something personal and allowing
  others to feel more connected to you rather
  than a concept.

- **A Self-assured Vibe:** As we mentioned in the
  previous chapter, having confidence is an
  important part of charisma. When you are
  confident, the vibe you give off to others shows
  that you believe in yourself at the core. This
  will cause people to be drawn to you because
  you have something that so many others don't.
  Learning how to be confident in yourself is a
  lifelong journey and can never happen
  overnight, but there is a quick trick that will
  help you get a boost in the moment next time
  you need one. It's called the posture of power:

  This posture involves standing up tall, bending

your knees slightly and standing with your feet below your shoulders. Then you want to reach your arms upward toward the sky as you smile and look up. Breathe deeply, attempting to fill your entire body and imagine that you are growing to expand and take up the whole room you are in. Hold this posture for 60 seconds to gain the mood-transforming benefits it has to offer. When the minute is over you will feel more charismatic and confident, ready to take on anything.

- **Know how to Ask Questions:** Since being charismatic is about making others feel important, you must know how to ask questions to get people to open up and engage with you. As soon as you notice that the person you are talking with seems to come upon a subject that they are excited by, you can encourage this train of thought by asking interested and open questions about it. For example, say you are talking to someone that mentions that they went fishing recently and they seem to light up at the memory of this. You can then proceed to ask how long they've been doing it, what their favorite part of the experience is, and more.

The best part about learning how to ask interested questions to others is that you will find that you receive interest back from them a lot easier than you would have before. This is because when we feel truly listened to, it's easier to respect someone and be interested in engaging with them and getting to know them better.

Each of the tips in this chapter will help you become a more charismatic, magnetic, and charming person to others. Keep in mind that this is not a journey that occurs overnight or instantly, but can be achieved with effort and practice. The more committed you are to becoming charismatic, the more likely you will be to reach that goal and stay there.

<u>You can Always Improve your Level of Charisma:</u>

Perhaps you are a person that already has some measure of charisma naturally. This doesn't mean that you can't benefit from the tips outlined above. Wherever we are in life, there is always room to move upward.

Chapter 4: How to Build Rapport

Rapport is defined as a state of being that is centered around understanding another person or group of people in a harmonious way that opens up easier and greater levels of communication. To say it another way, rapport means getting along with an individual or group of people by finding common ground with them, which opens up the line of communication and makes it more effective all around. There will be times when this happens on its own. You meet someone and click instantly, getting along perfectly without effort. This is how we choose our friends in life.

Is Rapport a Matter of Chance that we have No Control Over?

So, does this mean that it's all a matter of luck and we should simply hope for the best when it comes to rapport? Definitely not. While some may believe that you either get along with people or you don't, that is not the case. This quality is something that can be built up over time by learning how to find common interests with people, become more empathetic, and develop strong bonds.

This chapter will review methods for understanding what rapport is. It will also go over different methods for building it with new people, and how you can use it to benefit in life. Rapport matters a lot in personal and professional spheres alike, whether we are aware of its power or not. A manager is a lot more likely to choose a person that they sense will get along well with other employees. Relationships with other people, both in a romantic and platonic sense, are much simpler to forge and strengthen when both parties have a connection and understanding (or a high level of rapport) with each other.

Simple Factors to Keep in Mind about Rapport:

- **Body Language:** Someone who smiles a lot, looks people in the eye, and makes the effort to be courteous and polite to have a much better chance to build rapport with most anyone. This will make people like you a lot more often. Others are more prone to doing favors for others or treating them nicely if they are treated nicely first.

It's true that the first conversation you have

with a person can allow you to relax about interacting with them, but most building of rapport goes on independent of words and relies more on channels of communication that are unspoken. We maintain and start rapport beyond our conscious mind by matching up our signals to others, meaning the position of our body, where we look, the way we move, our tone of voice, and the expressions we show to the other person.

Observing two friends speaking with each other will show you how they match up to each other as they speak without even being aware of it. This is due to having strong rapport with each other. Rapport is built in an instinctive way since it is our natural way to defend against conflict (something that most people avoid at all costs, when possible).

We should always remember that using body language in an appropriate way is a huge foundational aspect of rapport. We instinctively pick up on and believe what we are told by the body language of another person, even though verbal communication may require more persuasion. If we claim one thing but our body language states another, the person we are talking to will believe what our body language is telling them. This means that creating rapport starts with adopting an open, relaxed, and welcoming body language posture.

- **Rapport is about "Matching up" with Others:** We have already reviewed why rapport is so important in relationships of all kinds, and why it should be the first thing you think about when approaching someone you hope to build a connection with. Creating rapport has a lot to do with matching up to others. A lot of people think that striking up a conversation with someone they don't know is a cause for anxiety. This can lead them to feel like they can't find the appropriate words or even become awkward with mannerisms, speech, or body language.

Being sure to create rapport at the very start while interacting with strangers will avoid this mishap and create an outcome that you will like a lot better, leading to positive possibilities. Regardless of how nervous or stressed out you feel at the thought of approaching someone, you must keep in mind that calmness is your best bet, and try to relax. You already get a head start with rapport by lowering your own tension, which the person will pick up on and respond to. You can practice deep breathing to get into a calm space before you begin the conversation.

Figure out the Best Icebreaking Methods:

When you meet a new person, these tips will aid you in reducing the nervousness you feel by letting you and the person you're speaking with relax and communicate in a more open and effective fashion:

- **Use Safe Conversation Topics at First:** When you are first approaching someone or trying to get to know them, you should make sure your choice of topic matter is not threatening in any way and is appropriate for small talk. This can mean you focus on experiences that you shared, how you got to the place you are, or the weather. Try not to talk about yourself too much and save personal or direct questions for later.

- **Seek Common Circumstances or Experiences**: Pay attention to what the person is talking about and search for circumstances or experiences that are shared. This will make it so you have more subject matter to discuss and more things to relate on in the beginning of the conversation.

- **Attempt to use Humor**: When you are interacting with a new person, humor is a great way to build rapport. When you laugh with someone, it creates an element of harmony to the conversation. This can involve making a joke related to the situation at hand or about yourself. You should, however, avoid making jokes about others since this can come off in the wrong way and turn people off from you.

- **Remember to Pay Attention to your Body Language**: You are constantly sending signals in a nonverbal way, whether you are aware of it or not. If you want to be better at building rapport, it pays to focus on this at least partially. You should try to make eye contact with the person you are speaking to more than half the time, without overdoing it. Lean toward them slightly in a relaxed fashion to show that you are listening and interested in what they are saying. You can also slightly mirror their posture if it makes sense at the time.

- **Relate with Empathy**: Show that you are capable of seeing what the other person has gone through or is trying to communicate. Keep in mind that rapport has a lot to do with relating through similarities or being on a similar level to the person. Learning how to come across as more empathetic will definitely help in this area.

- **Include, but don't Interrogate**: Since you might feel nervous talking to a new person, it's easy to go overboard with the questions and make it feel more like an interrogation than a back and forth conversation. Show that you care what they have to say without focusing on them too intently, since this can scare people off.

- **Match the Other Person's Words**: Although matching the body language of the person you are speaking to can help with rapport building, you can improve this even more by learning how to match the words of others. Clarifying what people say and reflecting it back to them is a useful way to show that you are listening. This will not only show you are paying attention but also create a chance to use phrases and words used by the person you're speaking to, emphasizing your similarity even more.

- **Pay Attention to your Tone of Voice**: How you speak is important, as well, in the way you build rapport with others. When someone is anxious or nervous, they have a tendency to rush through their words, coming off as stressed out or tense. We have the ability to change the pace, volume, and pitch of our voice at will to make what we are talking about more appealing. This will also help our speech to come across as friendlier and more relaxed. Try this by making an effort to speak more softly, slowly, and with a lower tone.

Keeping all of this in mind will make you have an easier time building rapport with others, leading to better opportunities, friendships, and relationships. In addition to the rapport building tips listed above, there are others you can try.

Behaviors for Building Rapport with Others:

- **Relaxed Posture and Gestures**: If you are speaking to someone and sitting down, you can appear more open by leaning forward toward them, leaving your legs and arms both uncrossed. This posture will show the person you are speaking to that you feel relaxed and comfortable, encouraging them to feel the same.

- **Friendly and Encouraging Motions**: When you listen to others, make sure you are nodding (but not too much), and displaying gestures and sounds that are encouraging. As someone talks, they subconsciously search for cues from the person they are talking to that shows that what they are saying is being heard and received.

- **Use their Name**: This should be done early on in the talk you are having with them. Not only will it help you remember their name but it will be seen as polite and likeable.

- **Summarize using Feedback**: You can clarify and reflect back your interpretation of what someone else is saying by summarizing their point and possibly adding open questions. This will create a chance for clearing up misunderstandings ahead of time. Also make a point to mention things later on in the conversation that mention what they have said earlier, proving that you were paying attention.

- **Forget about Stereotypes**: Try not to be judgmental toward whoever you are speaking with, since this will definitely get in the way of building rapport. Stay aware of any preconceived notions you might have of them and let them go before engaging in conversation.

- **Agreeing and Disagreeing Artfully**: When you agree with what another person is saying, you should state exactly why and say that you agree, building on the ideas they have said. If you must disagree, be sure to state the reason why first before saying that you don't agree.

- **Honesty is always Best**: When you aren't aware of the correct answer or have messed something up, own up to it. People respond well to honesty, and knowing how to admit mistakes will make others more likely to trust you. Be sure to always come across as a genuine person, using both verbal and visual methods for showing this.

- **Remember Simple Politeness**: Basic politeness in human interaction has to do with knowing how to compliment others, avoid conflict, and simply be nice. Don't underestimate the power of simple gestures.

Chapter 5: Self-Esteem

Self-esteem is the answer to how you feel about yourself. This is something that is learned throughout life and can be changed with effort. Your self-esteem is not something that is permanent and unchanging it. You can raise it at will, but should keep in mind that this is no simple task. Our self-esteem goes up in response to how often we face our own fears and accept lessons from tough experiences. For some, getting to the root of the issue may require therapy, but this chapter will cover some simple ways to begin improving your self-esteem.

The Negative Consequences of Low Self-Esteem:

Having a low level of self-esteem means that you hold yourself in negative regard, and this evaluation tends to show up when we go through some type of situation or circumstance that rubs us the wrong way, whether we are conscious of it or not. We then make the incident personal, going through emotional and physical responses to it. This can be very confusing, meaning that we react by engaging in ways that are self-defeating. When this occurs, we tend to act in ways that are impulsive and automatic, which can have negative effects in personal relationships, social life, and other aspects of existence.

Simple Ways to Raise your Self-Esteem over Time:

- **Take Care of Yourself:** This can involve quitting things that are bad for you (like smoking or junk food) and also cleaning up your mind by becoming more positive. You can join a group for this or read books on the topic to help you along the way.

- **Figure out your Triggers:** Everyone has triggers that can easily make them feel bad about themselves. This can be anything from receiving harmless criticism and taking it the wrong way to making a mistake and assuming that you are worthless because of it. Find out what your triggers are so you can avoid this automatic process.

If we view these triggers as a chance to gain more understanding about ourselves, we will be much better off. Next time a trigger pops up, try to stay conscious instead of automatically reacting in the same old way.

- **Try not to Take Things so Personally:** It's easy to feel bad about yourself if you think that everything is meant to harm you. Try, instead, to see things from the point of view of others. For example, if someone points out a mistake you made, they could just be trying to help.

- **Notice your Reactions:** Next time you see the tendency to want to overreact or take something personally, pause and pay attention. This will help you recognize patterns that can slow down the destructive habit of low self-esteem. You can also put your observation of your reaction into words to make it more real and slow down the impulse, but this is a lot more useful if you pair it with action instead of just passively noticing it.

- **Notice your Feelings:** A huge problem that leads to self-esteem complications is not being able to feel our emotions fully. Practice noticing your feelings in your body and fully embodying them, instead of trying to ignore them or suppress what they are trying to tell you. This will strengthen your sense of self as well as your intuition.

- **Stop Thinking in Black and White:** Try to adopt something known as thinking in options. Rather than assuming that everything has to be either this or that, think of the nuances involved in each situation. When you allow yourself to look at different options, you will be open to new ways of viewing problems in your life and finding better solutions.

Building healthy self-esteem is not a simple task, and takes effort and practice. However, by following along with the small suggestions listed above, you will be well on your way to becoming a lot healthier mentally and emotionally. When you have a high level of self-esteem, you can, as a consequence, become more charismatic and influential to other people. This will lead to healthier relationships, more friendships, and better opportunities in life.

Conclusion

Thank you again for downloading this book!

I hope this book was able to help you to define the word charisma for yourself, find out what it means to you, and see how it can apply to improving your relationship with yourself as well as others.

The next step is to follow the guidelines given in this book for developing your own charisma, becoming more confident, and building rapport with others. Soon, you will be on your way to becoming a master of social situations.

Finally, if you enjoyed this book, then I'd like to ask you for a favor, would you be kind enough to leave a review for this bo27ok on Amazon? It'd be greatly appreciated!

Thank you and good luck!